MINDFULNESS MEDITATION FOR BEGINNERS

A Step-by-Step Guide

Justin J. Williams

TABLE OF CONTENTS

CHAPTER 1

INTRODUCTION

In today's fast-paced and demanding world, it's easy to feel overwhelmed, stressed, and disconnected from our inner selves. The constant barrage of emails, notifications, and social media updates can leave us feeling distracted, anxious, and mentally exhausted. In such times, it's more important than ever to find ways to cultivate a sense of inner peace and well-being. That's where mindfulness meditation comes in.

Mindfulness meditation is a practice that has been around for thousands of years and is rooted in the Buddhist tradition. It involves intentionally focusing on the present moment, without judgment or distraction, and cultivating greater awareness and understanding of one's inner experience. Through mindfulness meditation, we learn to observe our thoughts, emotions, and physical sensations with curiosity and compassion, rather than getting lost in them or reacting to them impulsively.

In recent years, mindfulness meditation has gained widespread popularity in the Western world, as scientific research has shown it to be an effective tool for reducing stress, anxiety, and depression, and improving overall mental health and well-being. Studies have shown that regular mindfulness meditation practice can lead to changes in the brain that enhance emotional regulation, attention, and empathy.

But what exactly does mindfulness meditation involve? At its core, mindfulness meditation is a way of training the mind to focus on the present moment, rather than getting lost in thoughts or worries about the past or future. It often involves paying attention to the breath, the body, and the present moment with a sense of openness, curiosity, and acceptance.

There are many different types of mindfulness meditation, each with its unique focus and approach. Some forms of mindfulness meditation involve sitting quietly in a comfortable position and focusing on the breath, while others involve bringing mindfulness to everyday activities, such as walking, eating, or washing dishes. Regardless of the specific technique used, the goal of mindfulness meditation is to cultivate a sense of presence and awareness that can be carried into all aspects of life.

In this book, we'll be focusing on mindfulness meditation for beginners. Whether you're new to meditation or have tried it before with limited success, this book will provide you with a step-by-step guide to getting started with mindfulness meditation and developing a regular practice. We'll cover everything from setting up a comfortable meditation space to dealing with common challenges that may arise along the way. By the end of this book, you'll have the tools and knowledge you need to begin experiencing the many benefits of mindfulness meditation for yourself.

So why wait? Let's dive in and start exploring the world of mindfulness meditation together.

CHAPTER 2

THE BENEFITS OF MINDFULNESS MEDITATION FOR BEGINNERS

Mindfulness meditation is a powerful tool for cultivating greater awareness and presence in your daily life. When practiced regularly, it can help you develop a deeper understanding of your thoughts, emotions, and physical sensations, and cultivate greater compassion and empathy towards yourself and others.

Here are some of the key benefits of mindfulness meditation for beginners:

STRESS REDUCTION

Stress is a frequent sensation for many people in the fast-paced world of today. Whether it's due to work, relationships, or other sources of pressure, stress can have a significant impact on our physical and mental health. Mindfulness meditation is an effective tool for reducing stress levels by calming the nervous system and reducing the release of stress hormones like cortisol and adrenaline.

By bringing your attention to the present moment and cultivating an attitude of non-judgmental awareness towards your thoughts and emotions, you can develop a greater sense of calm and inner peace, even amid stressful situations. This can help you feel more centered and grounded, and better equipped to handle the challenges of everyday life.

IMPROVED MENTAL HEALTH

Mindfulness meditation is an effective tool for managing symptoms of depression, anxiety, and other mental health conditions. By developing greater awareness and understanding of your inner experience, you can learn to recognize patterns of thought and behavior that may be contributing to negative emotions and behaviors and develop more positive and adaptive coping strategies.

Research has also shown that mindfulness meditation can help reduce symptoms of PTSD and other trauma-related conditions,

and improve overall emotional well-being
and resilience.

INCREASED EMOTIONAL REGULATION

Mindfulness meditation can help you
develop greater emotional regulation by
teaching you to observe your thoughts and
emotions without judgment or attachment.

By cultivating a greater sense of
mindfulness and awareness, you can learn
to respond to difficult emotions with
greater equanimity and balance, rather
than reacting impulsively or getting caught
up in negative thought patterns.

This can be especially helpful in situations
where you might normally react with
anger, frustration, or other strong

emotions, allowing you to respond more skillfully and effectively to challenging situations.

IMPROVED FOCUS AND ATTENTION

Mindfulness meditation is a form of mental training that can improve your ability to focus and sustain attention. By practicing paying attention to the present moment, you can develop greater concentration and focus, which can be helpful in all areas of life, from work to relationships.

Research has shown that mindfulness meditation can also help improve working memory and cognitive flexibility, which can be especially beneficial for people in demanding or high-pressure jobs.

GREATER COMPASSION AND CONNECTION WITH OTHERS

Mindfulness meditation can help cultivate greater feelings of compassion and connection with others by helping you develop greater empathy and attunement to the experiences of those around you.

By developing greater awareness and understanding of your own inner experience, you can become more open and receptive to the experiences of others, and more willing to extend compassion and support to those in need.

Research has shown that mindfulness meditation can also help improve relationships by reducing feelings of hostility and promoting greater emotional intimacy and connection.

BETTER SLEEP

Mindfulness meditation can help promote better sleep by reducing stress and anxiety, which can interfere with sleep quality and duration. By cultivating greater awareness and presence in the present moment, you can learn to let go of racing thoughts and worries, and develop greater ease and relaxation in your body and mind.

Research has shown that mindfulness meditation can be an effective tool for improving sleep quality and reducing symptoms of insomnia and other sleep-related conditions.

These are just a few of the many benefits of mindfulness meditation for beginners. Whether you're looking to reduce stress, improve mental health, cultivate greater compassion and connection with others, or simply improve your overall well-being, mindfulness meditation can be a powerful tool for achieving your goals.

It's important to note that while mindfulness meditation can have many benefits, it's not a cure-all solution for every problem. It's important to seek out professional help if you're struggling with a serious mental health condition or other significant challenges in your life.

That said, mindfulness meditation can be a valuable complement to other forms of treatment and support, and can help you develop greater resilience and inner resources to cope with life's ups and downs.

In the following chapters, we'll explore some simple techniques for getting started with mindfulness meditation, and offer tips and guidance for building a sustainable and effective meditation practice. By incorporating mindfulness into your daily routine, you can start to experience the many benefits that this powerful practice has to offer.

CHAPTER 3

GETTING STARTED WITH MINDFULNESS MEDITATION

Mindfulness meditation can seem intimidating to those who are new to the practice, but it's quite simple to get started. By following some basic tips and techniques, you can develop a solid foundation for a sustainable and effective meditation practice.

FIND A QUIET AND COMFORTABLE SPACE

When starting your mindfulness meditation practice, it's important to find a quiet and comfortable space where you won't be interrupted. This could be a room in your home, a quiet corner of a park, or any other location where you feel relaxed and at ease.

Make sure to remove any potential distractions from your space, such as electronic devices, bright lights, or other people. This will allow you to fully focus on your meditation practice and cultivate a sense of inner stillness and calm.

START WITH SHORT SESSIONS

When starting with mindfulness meditation, it's important to start with short sessions of just a few minutes at a time. This allows you to build your skills gradually and avoid becoming overwhelmed or discouraged.

Try starting with just a few minutes of meditation each day, gradually increasing the length of your sessions as you become more comfortable with the practice. Even a few minutes of mindfulness meditation each day can have a significant impact on your mental health and overall well-being.

USE A TIMER

Using a timer can be a helpful tool for keeping track of your meditation sessions and avoiding the temptation to check the time or become distracted. You can use a timer on your phone, a dedicated meditation timer, or any other device that allows you to set a specific duration for your session.

When using a timer, choose a gentle, non-intrusive sound or tone that won't startle you out of your meditation practice. This could be a soft chime, a gentle bell, or any other soothing sound that helps you stay focused and present.

FOCUS ON YOUR BREATH

One of the simplest and most effective techniques for mindfulness meditation is to focus on your breath. This involves simply paying attention to the sensation of your breath as it flows in and out of your body, without trying to control or manipulate it in any way.

As you focus on your breath, try to notice the physical sensations of the air moving in and out of your nostrils, the expansion and contraction of your chest and abdomen, and any other sensations that arise in your body. If your thoughts start to stray, softly refocus on your breathing.

CULTIVATE AN ATTITUDE OF NON-JUDGMENTAL AWARENESS

When practicing mindfulness meditation, it's important to cultivate an attitude of non-judgmental awareness toward your thoughts, emotions, and physical sensations. This means observing your experience without trying to judge or change it in any way.

If you notice negative thoughts or emotions arising during your meditation practice, simply observe them without becoming attached to them or trying to suppress them. Instead, try to notice them with a sense of curiosity and openness, as if observing them from a distance.

By following these simple tips and techniques, you can start to develop a sustainable and effective mindfulness meditation practice. In the next chapter, we'll explore some additional techniques and strategies for taking your meditation practice to the next level.

CHAPTER 4

DEEPENING YOUR MINDFULNESS MEDITATION PRACTICE

Once you've established a regular mindfulness meditation practice, you may find that you're ready to deepen your practice and explore more advanced techniques. In this chapter, we'll explore some additional strategies for taking your mindfulness meditation practice to the next level.

BODY SCAN MEDITATION

Body scan meditation is a powerful technique for cultivating mindfulness and awareness of the physical sensations in your body. In this practice, you'll focus your attention on different parts of your body, noticing any physical sensations that arise without judgment or interpretation.

To practice body scan meditation, find a comfortable seated or lying position and begin by focusing your attention on your breath. Then, gradually bring your attention to different parts of your body, starting at your feet and moving up through your legs, torso, arms, and head.

As you focus on each part of your body, notice any physical sensations that arise, such as tension, tingling, or warmth. If you notice any discomfort or pain, simply observe it without judgment or interpretation, and gently move your attention to another part of your body.

LOVING-KINDNESS MEDITATION

Loving-kindness meditation is a powerful technique for cultivating feelings of love, compassion, and goodwill towards yourself and others. In this practice, you'll repeat a series of phrases or affirmations that express your wishes for well-being and happiness.

To practice loving-kindness meditation, find a comfortable seated position and begin by focusing your attention on your breath. Then, repeat the following phrases to yourself, either silently or aloud:

May I be happy.
May I be healthy.
May I be safe.
May I live with ease.

After repeating these phrases to yourself for a few minutes, begin to extend your wishes to others, starting with someone you love and care about deeply, and gradually expanding to include more difficult people in your life, and eventually all beings.

MINDFUL MOVEMENT

Mindful movement is a powerful technique for integrating mindfulness into your daily life and developing greater awareness of your body and physical sensations. In this practice, you'll move your body in a slow, deliberate, and mindful way, paying close attention to the physical sensations that arise.

To practice mindful movement, choose a simple movement, such as walking, stretching, or yoga, and move slowly and mindfully, paying attention to the physical sensations in your body. Notice the feeling of your feet on the ground, the movement of your muscles and joints, and any other physical sensations that arise.

As you practice mindful movement, try to maintain a sense of curiosity and openness, and avoid judging or interpreting your physical sensations. This can help you develop a deeper connection to your body and cultivate greater mindfulness in your daily life.

By incorporating these advanced techniques into your mindfulness meditation practice, you can deepen your connection to your body, cultivate greater awareness and compassion, and develop a greater sense of inner peace and well-being. In the next chapter, we'll explore some common challenges and obstacles that can arise during meditation practice and strategies for overcoming them.

CHAPTER 5

OVERCOMING OBSTACLES IN MINDFULNESS MEDITATION PRACTICE

Although mindfulness meditation can be a powerful tool for cultivating inner peace and well-being, it's not always easy to practice consistently. In this chapter, we'll explore some common challenges and obstacles that can arise during meditation practice and strategies for overcoming them.

PHYSICAL DISCOMFORT

One of the most common challenges of mindfulness meditation is physical discomfort. Sitting still for an extended period can be challenging, especially if you're not used to it. Additionally, physical sensations such as pain, stiffness, or tension can arise, which can be distracting and make it difficult to focus your attention.

To overcome physical discomfort, there are several strategies you can try. First, experiment with different meditation postures and props to find a comfortable position that works for you. You might try sitting on a cushion, using a meditation bench, or practicing in a chair with good back support.

Another strategy is to use mindfulness itself as a tool for managing physical discomfort. Rather than trying to push the discomfort away, simply notice it with curiosity and openness.

Observe the physical sensations in your body without judging them or trying to change them. This can help you develop a greater sense of acceptance and resilience in the face of physical discomfort.

MENTAL DISTRACTIONS

Another common obstacle in mindfulness meditation is mental distractions. Thoughts, emotions, and external stimuli can all pull your attention away from your meditation practice, making it difficult to stay focused and present.

To overcome mental distractions, one effective strategy is to use a mental "anchor" to help you stay focused. This might be your breath, a physical sensation in your body, or a repeated phrase or mantra.

Whenever your mind wanders, simply notice the distraction and gently bring your attention back to your anchor.

Another strategy is to practice "noting" your thoughts and emotions as they arise. Whenever you notice your mind wandering or becoming distracted, simply acknowledge the thought or emotion with a mental note, such as "thinking" or "feeling". Then, gently bring your attention back to your anchor.

RESISTANCE TO PRACTICE

Sometimes, even when we know that mindfulness meditation is good for us, we may find ourselves resistant to practicing regularly. We might feel bored, restless, or simply unmotivated to sit down and meditate.

To overcome resistance to practice, it can be helpful to explore the underlying reasons for your resistance. Are you feeling overwhelmed or stressed in other areas of your life? Are you struggling with self-doubt or negative self-talk? Once you've identified the root cause of your resistance, you can begin to develop strategies for addressing it.

One effective strategy is to set realistic goals and expectations for your meditation practice. Rather than trying to meditate for long periods every day, start small and gradually build up your practice over time.

You might try starting with just five or ten minutes of meditation each day, and gradually increasing the length of your sessions as you feel more comfortable and confident.

Another strategy is to practice self-compassion and kindness towards yourself. Remember that mindfulness meditation is a practice, and it's natural to have ups and downs along the way.

Rather than beating yourself up for missing a day of practice or struggling with distraction, simply notice your thoughts and emotions with curiosity and kindness, and gently guide yourself back to your meditation practice.

By developing strategies for overcoming common obstacles in mindfulness meditation practice, you can build a more sustainable and fulfilling meditation practice that supports your overall well-being and happiness.

In the next chapter, we'll explore some additional resources and tools for deepening your mindfulness meditation practice.

CHAPTER 6

DEEPENING YOUR MINDFULNESS MEDITATION PRACTICE

Now that you've established a regular mindfulness meditation practice and overcome some of the common obstacles that can arise, you may be interested in deepening your practice even further. In this chapter, we'll explore some additional resources and tools for taking your mindfulness meditation practice to the next level.

MINDFULNESS RETREATS

One powerful way to deepen your mindfulness meditation practice is to attend a mindfulness retreat. Retreats offer an opportunity to immerse yourself in your practice, away from the distractions and stresses of daily life.

They may range in length from a weekend to several weeks and can be held in a variety of settings, from wilderness retreat centers to urban meditation studios.

During a mindfulness retreat, you'll have the opportunity to practice meditation for extended periods, receive guidance and instruction from experienced teachers, and connect with a community of fellow meditators. Retreats can be a powerful way to deepen your practice and gain a new perspective on your life.

MINDFUL MOVEMENT PRACTICES

In addition to seated meditation, mindful movement practices such as yoga, tai chi, or qigong can be a powerful way to deepen your mindfulness practice. These practices combine gentle physical movement with breath awareness and present-moment awareness, helping to cultivate a deeper sense of embodied presence and relaxation.

Mindful movement practices can also help to increase physical flexibility, reduce stress and tension in the body, and improve overall physical and mental well-being. If you're interested in exploring mindful movement practices, consider taking a class at a local yoga studio or community center, or using online resources such as YouTube videos or mindfulness apps.

MINDFULNESS-BASED THERAPY

For those who are struggling with mental health challenges such as anxiety, depression, or chronic stress, mindfulness-based therapy can be a powerful tool for deepening your mindfulness meditation practice and gaining additional support and guidance.

Mindfulness-based therapy combines mindfulness meditation with cognitive-behavioral therapy (CBT) techniques, helping to identify and change negative patterns of thought and behavior. It can be effective for a wide range of mental health challenges and has been shown to improve overall well-being and quality of life.

If you're interested in exploring mindfulness-based therapy, consider finding a therapist who specializes in this approach or seeking out a mindfulness-based stress reduction program in your area.

MINDFULNESS-BASED ACTIVITIES

Finally, you can deepen your mindfulness meditation practice by incorporating mindfulness into other areas of your life. Mindfulness-based activities such as mindful eating, mindful walking, or mindful communication can help you cultivate a greater sense of present-moment awareness and connection in your daily life.

To incorporate mindfulness into your daily activities, start by choosing one or two activities that you engage in regularly, such as eating breakfast or walking to work. Before you begin the activity, take a few deep breaths and bring your attention to the present moment.

As you engage in the activity, notice the physical sensations, thoughts, and emotions that arise, without judgment or distraction.

By deepening your mindfulness meditation practice and incorporating mindfulness into other areas of your life, you can cultivate a greater sense of inner peace, resilience, and well-being. In the next chapter, we'll explore some tips and strategies for maintaining your mindfulness meditation practice over the long term.

CHAPTER 7

CONCLUSION

In this book, we've explored the basics of mindfulness meditation, including techniques for cultivating present-moment awareness, managing distracting thoughts, and developing greater self-awareness and compassion.

Whether you're a complete beginner or have some experience with meditation, we hope that you've found this guide to be informative and helpful.

Throughout this book, we've emphasized the importance of regular practice in developing mindfulness meditation skills. We've explored a variety of techniques for cultivating present-moment awareness, including breath meditation, body scan meditation, and loving-kindness meditation.

We've also discussed how to overcome common obstacles to meditation practice, such as restlessness, boredom, and self-doubt.

Additionally, we've explored how mindfulness meditation can benefit various aspects of your life, from reducing stress and anxiety to improving focus and productivity.

While mindfulness meditation can be challenging at times, it's also a powerful tool for improving well-being and living a more fulfilling life. By continuing to practice regularly, you can deepen your understanding of yourself and the world around you, as well as develop greater resilience and compassion.